Title: Fueling Performance: Nutrition Strategies for Athletes and Active Individuals

By

Sandy Yoder

Table of Contents

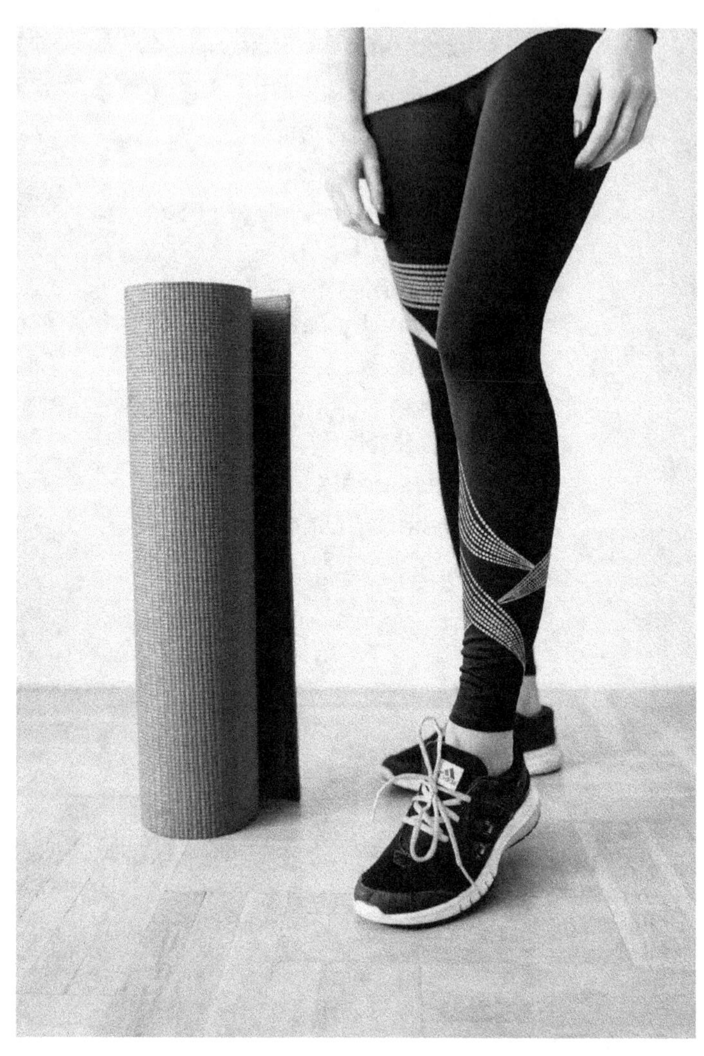

Chapter one

Introduction

Athletic prowess isn't just about training hard; it's also about feeding the body with the right fuel. Welcome to Fueling Performance: Nutrition Strategies for Athletes and Active Individuals. In this book, we embark on a journey to uncover the powerful correlation between what you eat and how well you perform in sports and other physical activities.

We'll explore how the food you consume directly influences your energy levels, endurance, strength, and overall athletic capabilities. From understanding the science behind macronutrients and micronutrients to tailoring nutrition for specific sports and delving into the realm of recovery and injury prevention, this book is your comprehensive guide to optimising performance through nutrition.

So, get ready to discover the secrets of peak performance, backed by scientific insights and practical advice. It's time to take control of your nutrition and unlock your full athletic potential.

A.Setting the Stage: The Crucial Role of Nutrition in Athletic Performance

Athletes often dedicate countless hours to training, pushing their limits, and honing their skills. Yet, what many overlook is the vital role that nutrition plays in elevating their performance from good to great.

Imagine your body as a high-performance machine: to function optimally, it requires the right kind of fuel. Nutrition serves as the foundation upon which athletic achievements are built. It's not merely about consuming calories but about strategically selecting nutrients that power your muscles, support recovery, and sustain endurance.

In this section, we'll delve into the profound impact nutrition has on an athlete's body and explore how the right dietary choices can sharpen focus, enhance strength, and significantly improve overall performance. Prepare to uncover the science behind this symbiotic relationship between nutrition and athletic prowess.

Understanding the Connection: Nutrition, Energy, and Performance

Nutrition isn't just about filling up; it's about fueling your body with the precise elements it needs to thrive. At its core, nutrition serves as the primary source of energy for the body's intricate machinery, enabling athletes to reach peak performance.

This section illuminates the interplay between nutrition, energy levels, and athletic performance. We'll unravel the mechanisms by which carbohydrates, proteins, and fats act as the body's fuel, providing the energy necessary for optimal physical exertion. Moreover, we'll explore how micronutrients like vitamins and minerals contribute to energy metabolism and overall performance enhancement.

Prepare to uncover the secrets behind how the right nutrition doesn't just sustain energy but maximises it, allowing athletes to push boundaries, exceed limits, and achieve their personal best.

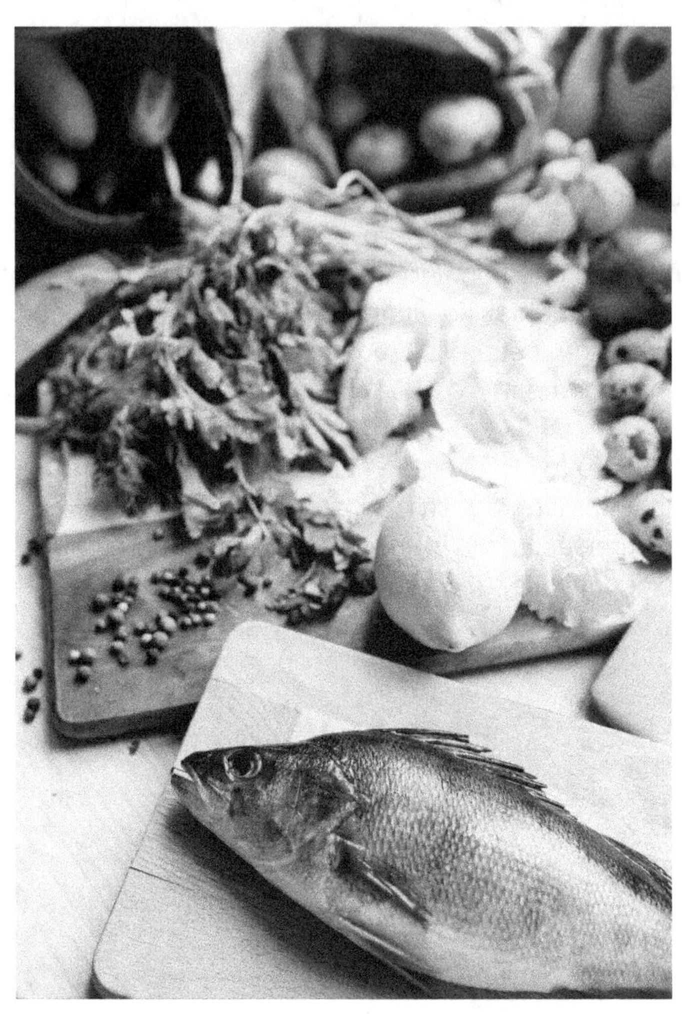

Chapter Two

The Science Behind Nutrition and Performance

I. **Macronutrients**: Fueling the Body for Optimal Performance
A. **Carbohydrates**: The Primary Energy Source
1. Exploring the Role of Carbohydrates in Energy Production
2. Understanding Glycogen Stores and Endurance

B. **Proteins: Building Blocks for Strength and Recovery**
1. Protein's Crucial Role in Muscle Repair and Growth
2. Protein Timing and Distribution for Athletic Performance

C. **Fats: Balancing Energy and Endurance**
1. Differentiating Between Types of Fats and Their Impact
2. Fat Utilisation in Long-Term Energy Expenditure

II. **Micronutrients**: Vitamins and Minerals for Enhanced Performance
A. Importance of Key Micronutrients
1. Examining Vitamins and Their Role in Energy Metabolism
2. Minerals' Contribution to Muscle Function and Recovery

B. **Micronutrient Deficiencies and Performance Impact**
1. Effects of Deficient Micronutrients on Athletic Performance
2. Strategies to Address and Prevent Micronutrient Deficiencies

Through a comprehensive exploration of macronutrients and micronutrients, this section unveils the intricate science governing how these elements serve as the building blocks and catalysts for an athlete's performance. By understanding the nuanced roles of carbohydrates, proteins, fats, vitamins, and minerals, athletes can optimise their nutrition to propel their athletic capabilities to new heights.

1.Macronutrients: Fueling the Body for Optimal Performance
I. Carbohydrates: The Primary Energy Source
Carbohydrates stand as the body's preferred and most efficient fuel source for high-intensity activities. This section delves into:

A. Exploring the Role of Carbohydrates in Energy Production
- Understanding the Glycemic Index and Its Impact on Performance
- Timing Carbohydrate Intake for Enhanced Energy Availability

B. **Understanding Glycogen Stores and Endurance**
- **Glycogen Depletion**: Effects on Endurance and Performance
- Strategies for Glycogen Replenishment and Prolonged Endurance

II. **Proteins: Building Blocks for Strength and Recovery**
Proteins serve as the fundamental building blocks for muscle repair, growth, and recovery. This part illuminates:

A. Protein's Crucial Role in Muscle Repair and Growth
- Protein Quality and its Influence on Muscle Protein Synthesis
- Protein Requirements for Different Athletes and Activity Levels

B. **Protein Timing and Distribution for Athletic Performance**
- Optimal Timing of Protein Intake for Recovery and Performance
- Protein Distribution Throughout the Day for Sustained Muscle Health

III. **Fats: Balancing Energy and Endurance**
Fats play a multifaceted role in providing sustained energy and supporting endurance. This section addresses:

A. **Differentiating Between Types of Fats and Their Impact**

- **Understanding Healthy vs. Unhealthy Fats for Athletic** Performance

- Fat Adaptation and its Role in Long-Term Energy Expenditure

B. **Fat Utilisation in Long-Term Energy Expenditure**
- Maximising Fat Utilisation for Endurance Activities
- Incorporating Healthy Fats for Sustained Energy Levels

By dissecting the roles and optimal utilisation of carbohydrates, proteins, and fats, athletes gain a nuanced understanding of how to strategically employ these macronutrients to elevate their athletic performance.

Carbohydrates: The Primary Energy Source

Carbohydrates stand as the body's foremost energy source, crucial for sustaining high-intensity physical activities. This section delves into:

1. **Exploring the Role of Carbohydrates in Energy Production**
Glycemic Index and Performance: Understanding how different carbohydrate sources impact energy

levels and endurance during workouts or competitions.

Timing Carbohydrate Intake: Strategies for optimising

carbohydrate consumption pre-, during, and post-exercise to enhance energy availability and performance.

2. Understanding Glycogen Stores and Endurance

Glycogen Depletion Effects: Exploring how depleted glycogen stores affect endurance and strategies to mitigate its impact on athletic performance.

Replenishing Glycogen: Techniques and timelines for efficiently replenishing glycogen stores to sustain endurance and prevent fatigue during prolonged activities.

This section equips athletes with insights into harnessing carbohydrates effectively, ensuring adequate energy stores for optimal performance and prolonged endurance during training and competitions.

Proteins: Building Blocks for Strength and Recovery

Proteins play a pivotal role in muscle repair, growth, and overall recovery, essential for athletes aiming to maximise their performance. This section offers comprehensive insights into:

1. Protein's Crucial Role in Muscle Repair and Growth

Muscle Protein Synthesis: Understanding how proteins facilitate muscle repair and the synthesis of new muscle tissue after physical exertion.

Quality of Protein: Exploring the significance of different protein sources and their impact on muscle protein synthesis and recovery.

2. Protein Timing and Distribution for Athletic Performance

Optimal Timing for Recovery: Strategies for consuming proteins post-exercise to enhance recovery and muscle repair.

Daily Distribution: Guidelines for distributing protein intake across meals to sustain muscle health and facilitate ongoing repair and growth.

This section empowers athletes with knowledge about leveraging proteins strategically, ensuring they aid in muscle repair, growth, and recovery, thereby optimising overall athletic performance.

Fats: Balancing Energy and Endurance

Fats serve as a multifaceted resource in providing sustained energy and supporting an athlete's endurance. This section illuminates:

1. Differentiating Between Types of Fats and Their Impact

Healthy vs. Unhealthy Fats: Understanding the distinction between different fat types and their respective effects on athletic performance and overall health.

Fat Adaptation: Exploring the concept of fat adaptation and its role in enhancing long-term energy expenditure and endurance.

2. Fat Utilisation in Long-Term Energy Expenditure

Maximising Fat Utilisation: Strategies to optimise the utilisation of fats as a fuel source during endurance activities.

Incorporating Healthy Fats: Guidelines on incorporating healthy fats into the diet to maintain sustained energy levels and support overall performance.

By dissecting the roles and nuances of different fats, athletes gain insights into utilising fats optimally for sustained energy, endurance, and overall athletic performance.

B. Micronutrients: Vitamins and Minerals for Enhanced Performance

Micronutrients, namely vitamins and minerals, are instrumental in optimising athletic performance. This section explores their significance:

1. **Importance of Key** Micronutrients
Vitamins in Energy Metabolism: Unveiling how vitamins contribute to energy production, cellular function, and overall athletic performance.

Minerals and Muscle Function:

Understanding the role of minerals in muscle contraction, recovery, and performance enhancement.

2. **Micronutrient Deficiencies and Performance Impact**
Effects of Deficiencies: Exploring how deficiencies in key micronutrients can impair athletic performance and strategies to mitigate these effects.

Prevention Strategies: Tips and methods to ensure athletes maintain adequate levels of vitamins and minerals to optimise performance and recovery.

This section equips athletes with knowledge about harnessing the power of micronutrients to elevate their performance, focusing on the essential role these elements play in energy metabolism, muscle function, and overall well-being.

1. Importance of Key Micronutrients

The significance of key micronutrients, such as vitamins and minerals, cannot be overstated in the context of athletic performance:

Vitamins in Energy Metabolism
Energy Production: Various B vitamins (B1, B2, B3, B6, B12) aid in converting food into energy, crucial for sustaining endurance and performance during workouts or competitions.

Antioxidant Defence: Vitamins C and E act as antioxidants, protecting cells from oxidative stress induced by intense physical activity, thereby supporting overall recovery.

Minerals and Muscle Function
Electrolyte Balance: Minerals like sodium, potassium, calcium, and magnesium maintain electrolyte balance, crucial for muscle contraction, nerve function, and hydration.

Oxygen Transport: Iron is pivotal in oxygen transportation, as it's a core component of haemoglobin in red blood cells, enhancing oxygen delivery to muscles for optimal performance.

Understanding and ensuring adequate intake of these micronutrients is fundamental for athletes as they directly impact energy production, muscle function, recovery, and overall athletic performance.

2. Micronutrient Deficiencies and Performance Impact

Micronutrient deficiencies can significantly impact an athlete's performance:

Effects of Deficiencies:

Reduced Energy Levels:

Insufficient B vitamins can hamper energy production, leading to fatigue and decreased stamina during workouts or competitions.

Muscle Weakness and Cramps: Deficiencies in minerals like calcium, potassium, or magnesium can result in muscle weakness, cramps, and impaired muscle function, affecting overall performance.

Decreased Immunity: Inadequate intake of vitamins C and E may compromise the immune system, making athletes more susceptible to illnesses that could disrupt training schedules.

Prevention Strategies:
Balanced Diet: Ensuring a varied and balanced diet rich in fruits, vegetables, lean proteins, and whole grains to cover a wide spectrum of essential vitamins and minerals.

Supplementation, if Necessary:

Consideration of supplements under the guidance of a healthcare professional to address specific deficiencies that diet alone may not adequately cover.

Addressing and preventing micronutrient deficiencies is crucial for athletes to maintain peak performance, avoid fatigue, support muscle function, and fortify their immune system against potential disruptions to their training regimens

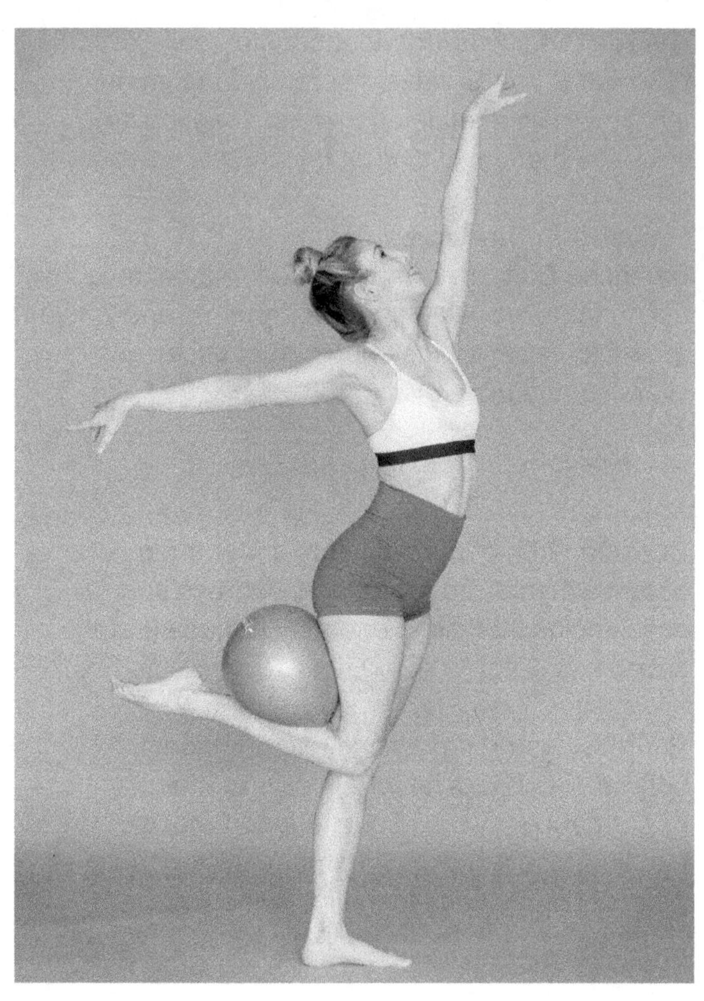

Chapter Three

III. **Tailoring Nutrition for Specific Sports and Activities**

Athletes engaged in different sports and activities have unique nutritional needs to optimise their performance. This section explores tailored strategies for various types of athletic pursuits:

A. **Endurance Sports**: Strategies for Sustained Energy
Nutritional Needs: Examining the specific requirements for endurance athletes like runners, cyclists, and triathletes, emphasising sustained energy and endurance.

Hydration and Electrolyte Balance: Addressing the crucial role of hydration and electrolyte replenishment during prolonged activities to prevent dehydration and maintain performance.

B. **Strength and Power Sports**: Building Muscle, Enhancing Recovery
Protein Requirements: Focusing on increased protein needs for athletes engaged in strength and power sports to support muscle repair and growth.

Recovery Nutrition: Highlighting the significance of post-workout nutrition and recovery strategies to optimise muscle recovery and prevent injury.

C. **Team Sports**: Optimising Performance and Recovery
Intermittent High-Intensity Activity: Understanding the nutritional demands of team sports that involve bursts of high-intensity activities, emphasising fueling strategies for optimal performance.

Pre- and Post-Game Nutrition:

 Addressing the importance of pre-game fueling and post-game recovery nutrition for sustained energy and muscle repair.

Tailoring nutrition based on the specific demands of each sport or activity ensures athletes receive the appropriate macronutrients, hydration, and timing of meals to support their unique physical requirements, enhance performance, and aid in recovery.

A. Endurance Sports: Strategies for Sustained Energy

Athletes engaged in endurance activities such as running, cycling, and triathlons require sustained energy to perform at their best. This section delves into tailored nutritional strategies for these athletes:

1. **Nutritional Needs for Endurance Athletes**
Carbohydrate Loading: Exploring carbohydrate-loading techniques to maximise glycogen stores before endurance events, optimising fuel availability.

Fueling During Exercise:

Strategies for consuming carbohydrates during long-duration activities to maintain energy levels and prevent fatigue or "hitting the wall."

2. **Hydration and Electrolyte Balance**
Fluid Replacement: Emphasising the importance of adequate hydration before, during, and after endurance activities to maintain performance and prevent dehydration.

Electrolyte Management:

Addressing the role of electrolytes like sodium, potassium, and magnesium in maintaining fluid balance and preventing cramping.

Tailoring nutrition for endurance athletes involves optimising carbohydrate intake for sustained energy, ensuring proper hydration, and managing electrolyte levels to support prolonged performance and prevent fatigue during endurance events.

1. **Nutritional Needs for Runners, Cyclists, and Triathletes**

Each endurance sport—running, cycling, and triathlons—has specific nutritional demands to sustain performance. Here's a breakdown of their nutritional needs:

1. **Runners** Carbohydrate Emphasis:

Focus on consuming carbohydrates to sustain energy levels during long-distance runs.

Hydration: Ensuring adequate fluid intake to prevent dehydration, especially during extended runs in varying climates.

2. **Cyclists** Carbohydrate Loading:

Optimising glycogen stores through carbohydrate-rich diets to support extended periods of cycling.

Electrolyte Balance: Managing electrolytes during long rides to prevent muscle cramps and maintain performance.

3. **Triathletes**
Transition Nutrition: Strategies to navigate transitions between swim, bike, and run segments

with appropriate fueling without gastrointestinal distress.

 Ensuring consistent hydration and fueling strategies across all segments of the triathlon for sustained energy.

Understanding the nuances of nutritional needs specific to running, cycling, and triathlons enables athletes to tailor their dietary intake effectively, optimising performance and endurance for their chosen endurance sport.

2. Hydration and Electrolyte Balance

Importance of Hydration:
Fluid Balance: Maintaining adequate hydration levels to support overall bodily functions, especially during strenuous physical activity.

Performance Impact: Dehydration can lead to decreased performance, fatigue, impaired cognitive function, and increased risk of heat-related illnesses.

Strategies for Optimal Hydration:
Pre-Exercise Hydration: Ensuring athletes are adequately hydrated before starting any physical activity.

During Exercise: Implementing hydration strategies by consuming fluids regularly, considering the duration and intensity of the activity.

Electrolyte Balance:Role of Electrolytes: Understanding the significance of electrolytes (sodium, potassium, magnesium) in maintaining fluid balance, nerve function, and muscle contraction.

Replenishment during Exercise:

Addressing the need to replenish electrolytes lost through sweat during prolonged activities, especially in hot or humid conditions.

Balancing hydration and electrolytes is critical for athletes to sustain performance, prevent dehydration-related complications, and optimise their endurance during workouts and competitions. Tailoring hydration strategies based on individual needs and environmental conditions is key to achieving peak athletic performance.

B. Strength and Power Sports: Building Muscle, Enhancing Recovery

Athletes engaged in strength and power-focused sports require specific nutritional strategies to support muscle development and facilitate effective recovery. This section addresses their unique needs:

1. Protein Requirements for Muscle Development

Increased Protein Intake: Emphasising higher protein intake to support muscle repair, growth, and adaptation in response to strength training.

Protein Quality: Focusing on high-quality protein sources to maximise muscle protein synthesis and optimise recovery.

2. Recovery Nutrition for Muscle Repair

Post-Workout Nutrition: Highlighting the importance of immediate post-exercise nutrition to replenish glycogen stores and initiate muscle recovery.

Nutrient Timing: Understanding the significance of timing protein and carbohydrate intake to facilitate muscle repair and minimise muscle breakdown.

For athletes involved in strength and power sports, optimising protein intake and post-exercise nutrition is crucial to support muscle growth, enhance recovery, and improve overall performance during intense training sessions and competitions.

In strength and power-focused sports, meeting elevated protein needs is crucial for optimal muscle development. Here's an in-depth look at this critical aspect:

1. Increased Protein Intake for Muscle Growth Elevated Protein Requirements: Understanding the heightened need for protein intake to support muscle repair and growth induced by strength training.

Ideal Protein Sources: Exploring sources of high-quality proteins like lean meats, dairy, eggs, legumes, and supplements to meet these increased requirements.

2. Protein Quality and Muscle Protein Synthesis Essential Amino Acids: Emphasising the importance of essential amino acids in protein sources to stimulate muscle protein synthesis optimally.

Timing and Distribution: Considering both the timing and distribution of protein intake across meals to maximise muscle repair and growth throughout the day.

Understanding and meeting these increased protein demands strategically can significantly impact muscle development and recovery, essential components for athletes engaged in strength and power-based sports aiming for peak performance.

2. Recovery Nutrition and Injury Prevention

Ensuring proper recovery nutrition is essential for athletes to facilitate muscle repair, prevent injuries, and sustain optimal performance. Here's a breakdown:

1. Post-Workout Nutrition for Recovery

Glycogen Replenishment: Focusing on carbohydrate intake post-exercise to replenish glycogen stores and aid in muscle recovery.

Protein for Repair: Emphasising the importance of consuming protein shortly after workouts to initiate muscle repair and growth.

2. Injury Prevention Strategies

Nutritional Support for Tissue Health: Exploring nutrients like vitamins C and D, omega-3 fatty acids, and antioxidants that support tissue health and injury prevention.

Balanced Diet for Overall Health:

Highlighting the significance of a balanced diet rich in nutrients to support a robust immune system and overall body resilience.

Implementing effective recovery nutrition strategies not only aids in muscle repair and growth but also plays a vital role in preventing injuries, enhancing an athlete's overall health, and ensuring sustained performance over time.

C. **Team Sports: Optimising Performance and Recovery**

Athletes engaged in team sports require tailored nutrition strategies to support their intermittent high-intensity activities and promote efficient recovery. Here's an overview:

1. **Intermittent High-Intensity Activity Fueling Strategies**: Addressing the need for energy-dense meals and snacks to support quick bursts of energy required during the game.

Carbohydrate Emphasis:

Focusing on carbohydrate-rich options to replenish energy stores for repeated bursts of high-intensity effort.

2. **Pre- and Post-Game Nutrition**

Pre-Game Fueling: Highlighting the importance of pre-game meals to optimise energy levels and performance without causing discomfort during play.

Post-Game Recovery:

Emphasising quick recovery nutrition after matches to replenish glycogen stores, repair muscle damage, and support recovery.

Tailoring nutrition to meet the demands of intermittent high-intensity activities in team sports ensures athletes have the necessary energy and resources to perform optimally during games while facilitating efficient recovery afterward, enhancing overall performance and reducing the risk of injury or fatigue.

1. Fueling for Intermittent High-Intensity Activity

In team sports involving intermittent bursts of high-intensity efforts, optimal nutrition is crucial to sustain energy levels throughout the game. Here's how athletes can fuel effectively:

1. **Energy-Dense Meals and Snacks**
Complex Carbohydrates: Including complex carbohydrates like whole grains, fruits, and vegetables in meals for sustained energy release.

 Incorporating easily digestible snacks like fruits, energy bars, or sports drinks for immediate energy boosts during breaks.

2. Carbohydrate Emphasis

Fueling Before Activity: Consuming moderate amounts of carbohydrates pre-activity to ensure adequate glycogen stores for bursts of high-intensity efforts.

Replenishment During Breaks:

Utilising halftime or breaks to replenish glycogen stores with carbohydrate-rich snacks or drinks to sustain energy levels.

Adopting a nutrition plan that prioritises carbohydrates, both before and during the game, supports athletes in maintaining their energy reserves, enabling them to perform optimally during the intermittent high-intensity phases characteristic of team sports.

2. Pre- and Post-Game Nutrition Strategies

Strategic nutrition before and after games is crucial for optimising performance and supporting recovery. Here's a breakdown of effective strategies:

1. Pre-Game Fueling

Balanced Meal: Consuming a balanced meal 2-3 hours before the game, consisting of carbohydrates, lean proteins, and healthy fats for sustained energy.

Pre-Game Snack: Having a smaller snack 30-60 minutes before the game, focusing on easily digestible carbohydrates to top up energy levels without causing discomfort.

2. Post-Game Recovery

Immediate Refuelling: Consuming a blend of carbohydrates and proteins within 30-60 minutes post-game to replenish glycogen stores and initiate muscle repair.

Hydration: Prioritising hydration by replenishing fluids lost during the game, ideally including electrolytes for optimal recovery.

Implementing effective pre-game fueling and post-game recovery strategies ensures athletes have the energy and nutrients needed to perform at their best during the game while kick-starting the recovery process to minimise muscle damage and fatigue afterward.

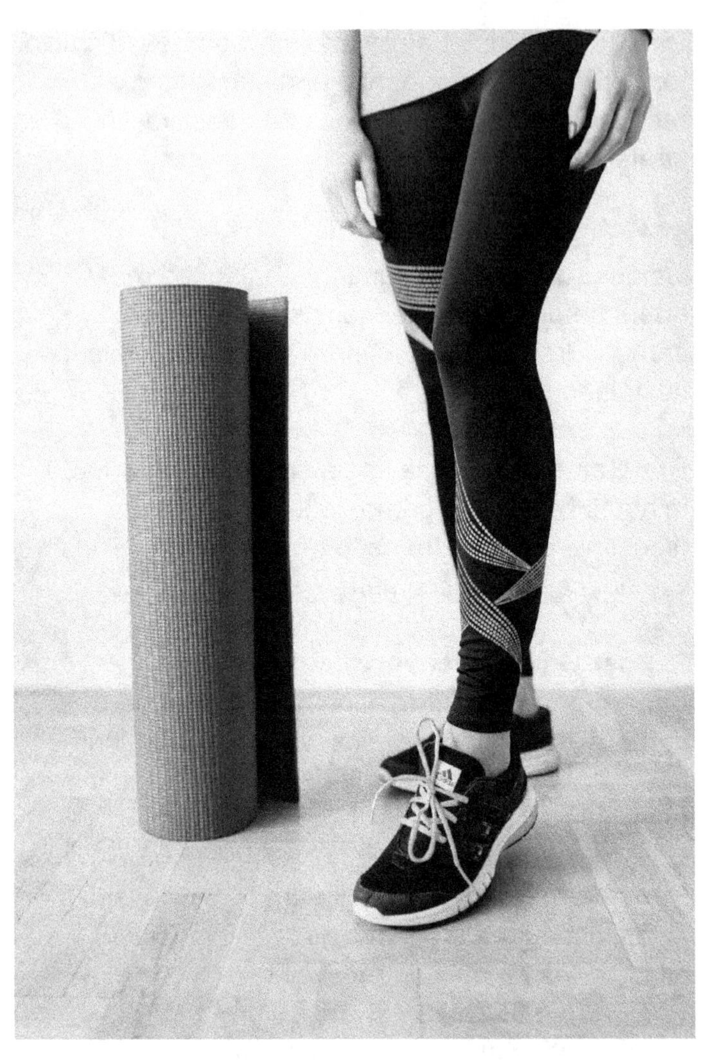

Chapter Four

IV. Nutrition for Optimal Recovery and Injury Prevention

Proper nutrition plays a vital role in both recovery post-exercise and in reducing the risk of injuries for athletes. Here's how nutrition can aid in these aspects:

1. Recovery Nutrition
Post-Exercise Fueling: Consuming a blend of carbohydrates and proteins within an hour post-exercise to replenish glycogen stores and initiate muscle repair.

Hydration: Ensuring adequate fluid intake to replace lost fluids and electrolytes during exercise, aiding in recovery and reducing the risk of muscle cramps.

2. Injury Prevention Strategies
Nutrient-Rich Diet: Adopting a balanced and nutrient-rich diet comprising vitamins, minerals, and antioxidants to support tissue health and aid in injury prevention.

Omega-3 Fatty Acids:

Incorporating sources of omega-3 fatty acids to reduce inflammation and support joint health, potentially reducing injury risks.

By focusing on proper post-exercise nutrition and maintaining a diet rich in essential nutrients, athletes can expedite their recovery process, reduce muscle soreness, and fortify their bodies against injuries, contributing to their overall performance and well-being.

A. Importance of Recovery Nutrition

Recovery nutrition holds immense importance for athletes due to its significant impact on various aspects of their performance and overall well-being:

1. **Muscle Repair and Growth**
Muscle Recovery: Adequate post-exercise nutrition with the right balance of carbohydrates and proteins initiates muscle repair, aiding in the recovery process after strenuous workouts or competitions.

2. Glycogen ReplenishmentEnergy Restoration:

Consuming carbohydrates post-exercise helps replenish glycogen stores, ensuring athletes have the energy reserves necessary for subsequent training sessions or competitions.

3. Reducing Fatigue and SorenessReduced Muscle Fatigue:

Proper recovery nutrition minimises muscle fatigue, allowing athletes to perform consistently at high levels.

Less Soreness: Effective post-exercise nutrition can also reduce muscle soreness, enabling athletes to recover faster between training sessions or games.

4. Injury Prevention

Tissue Repair: Nutrition rich in vitamins, minerals, and antioxidants supports tissue health, potentially reducing the risk of injuries.

Optimising recovery nutrition is fundamental for athletes as it accelerates the recovery process, reduces fatigue, aids in muscle repair and growth, and contributes significantly to their overall performance and injury prevention strategies.

Nutritional strategies play a crucial role in both preventing injuries and aiding in the healing process. Here are key approaches:

1. **Nutrient-Rich Diet for Injury Prevention Vitamins and Minerals:** Consuming a diverse range of fruits, vegetables, and whole grains to ensure adequate intake of vitamins (like C, D, and E) and minerals (such as calcium, magnesium, and zinc) that support tissue health and immune function, reducing the risk of injuries.

Omega-3 Fatty Acids:

Including sources of omega-3 fatty acids (like fatty fish, flaxseeds, chia seeds) to reduce inflammation and support joint health, potentially lowering the risk of certain injuries.

2. **Nutrition for Healing and RecoveryProtein-Rich Diet:**

 Ensuring sufficient protein intake to support tissue repair and aid in the healing process after an injury.

Caloric Sufficiency: Maintaining a balanced diet with adequate calories to support the body's increased energy needs during the healing phase.

Hydration: Staying properly hydrated to aid in overall recovery, tissue repair, and to prevent complications during the healing process.

By focusing on a nutrient-rich diet, adequate protein intake, and ensuring proper hydration, athletes can significantly contribute to injury prevention, promote faster healing, and improve overall recovery outcomes.

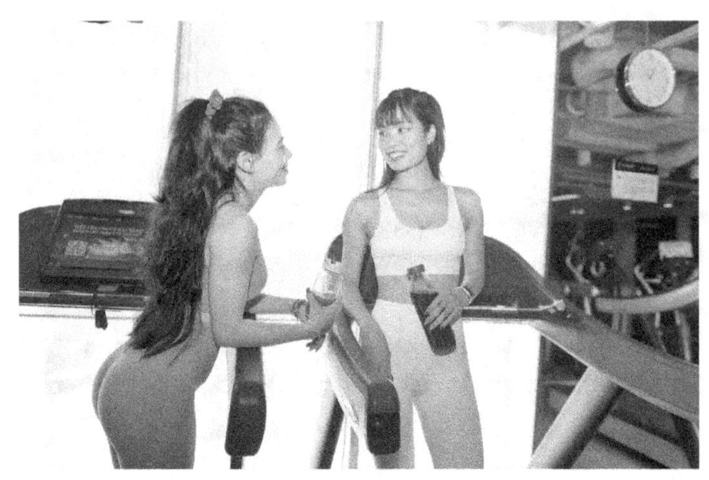

Chapter Five

V. Special Considerations and Advanced Strategies

Certainly, in the realm of sports nutrition, there are several special considerations and advanced strategies that athletes may explore to optimise their performance:

1. **Nutrition for Special Populations**
Youth Athletes: Tailoring nutritional needs for young athletes to support growth, development, and performance without compromising health.

Older Athletes:

Addressing specific nutritional needs for older athletes, focusing on maintaining muscle mass, bone health, and optimising recovery.

2. **Supplements**: Understanding Their Role and Risks
Supplement Use: Exploring the potential benefits and risks of various supplements commonly used by athletes, emphasising informed and cautious supplementation.

 Considering personalised supplementation needs based on deficiencies or specific performance goals under professional guidance.

3. **Mental Performance**: Influence of Nutrition on Focus and Cognitive Function
Brain Health: Exploring the impact of nutrition on brain function, focus, and cognitive abilities during training and competition.

Nutritional Strategies:

Implementing specific diets or nutrients that may enhance mental clarity, focus, and overall cognitive performance.

These considerations delve deeper into the nuanced aspects of sports nutrition, addressing individual needs, supplement use, and the relationship between nutrition and mental performance, enabling athletes to optimise their overall well-being and athletic capabilities.

A. **Nutrition for Special Populations** (e.g., youth athletes, older athletes)

Absolutely, tailoring nutrition for special populations, such as youth and older athletes, is crucial to meet their unique needs:

1. Nutrition for Youth Athletes

Balanced Diet: Emphasising the importance of a well-rounded diet rich in nutrients to support growth, development, and sustained energy for training and competitions.

Hydration:

Educating young athletes on proper hydration habits to maintain performance and prevent dehydration during activities.

2. Nutrition for Older Athletes

Protein Intake: Highlighting the significance of increased protein intake for maintaining muscle mass and strength in older athletes.

Calcium and Vitamin D:

Focusing on calcium and vitamin D intake to support bone health and reduce the risk of fractures or injuries.

Customising nutrition plans for these special populations ensures they receive the essential nutrients required for their respective life stages, enabling them to perform optimally while safeguarding their health and well-being.

B. Supplements: Understanding Their Role and Risks

Understanding supplements, their roles, and potential risks is crucial for athletes considering their use:

1. Role of Supplements

Fill Nutritional Gaps: Supplements can help fill nutritional gaps when athletes struggle to meet their dietary needs through food alone.

Performance Enhancement:

Some supplements claim to boost performance, aid recovery, or support specific aspects like muscle growth or endurance.

2. Risks and Considerations

Regulatory Oversight: Many supplements lack strict regulation or quality control, leading to potential contamination or inaccuracies in labelling.

Individual Responses:

Supplements may have varying effects on individuals, and their efficacy can differ based on genetic factors and overall health.

3. **Informed and Cautious Approach**

Professional Guidance: Seeking advice from qualified sports nutritionists or healthcare providers before incorporating supplements into their regiment

Testing and Research:

Ensuring supplements are batch-tested for quality and safety, and relying on peer-reviewed research to validate their efficacy.

By approaching supplements with caution, seeking professional advice, and being discerning about their quality and efficacy, athletes can mitigate potential risks and optimise the benefits that supplements might offer within their training and performance goals.

C. Mental Performance: The Influence of Nutrition on Focus and Cognitive Function

Nutrition plays a significant role in mental performance, focus, and cognitive function for athletes. Here's how:

1. Impact of Nutrition on Brain Health

Nutrient Influence: Certain nutrients like omega-3 fatty acids, antioxidants, vitamins, and minerals directly impact brain health and function.

Energy Demands: The brain requires a substantial amount of energy; hence, a balanced diet ensures an adequate supply for optimal cognitive function.

2. Nutritional Strategies for Mental Clarity and Focus

Hydration: Proper hydration supports cognitive function and prevents mental fatigue during training and competitions.

Balanced Macronutrients:

Consuming balanced meals with carbohydrates, proteins, and fats aids in sustained energy levels, crucial for mental alertness.

3. Advanced Nutritional Approaches

Specific Diets: Certain diets (e.g., Mediterranean diet, DASH diet) rich in fruits, vegetables, whole grains, and healthy fats show positive correlations with cognitive health.

Supplements for Brain Health:

Some supplements like omega-3 fatty acids or specific antioxidants may support cognitive function, but their effects can vary among individuals.

Optimising nutrition for mental performance involves providing the brain with the necessary nutrients for optimal function, hydration, and considering advanced dietary approaches that may positively impact cognitive health and focus for athletes during training and competition.

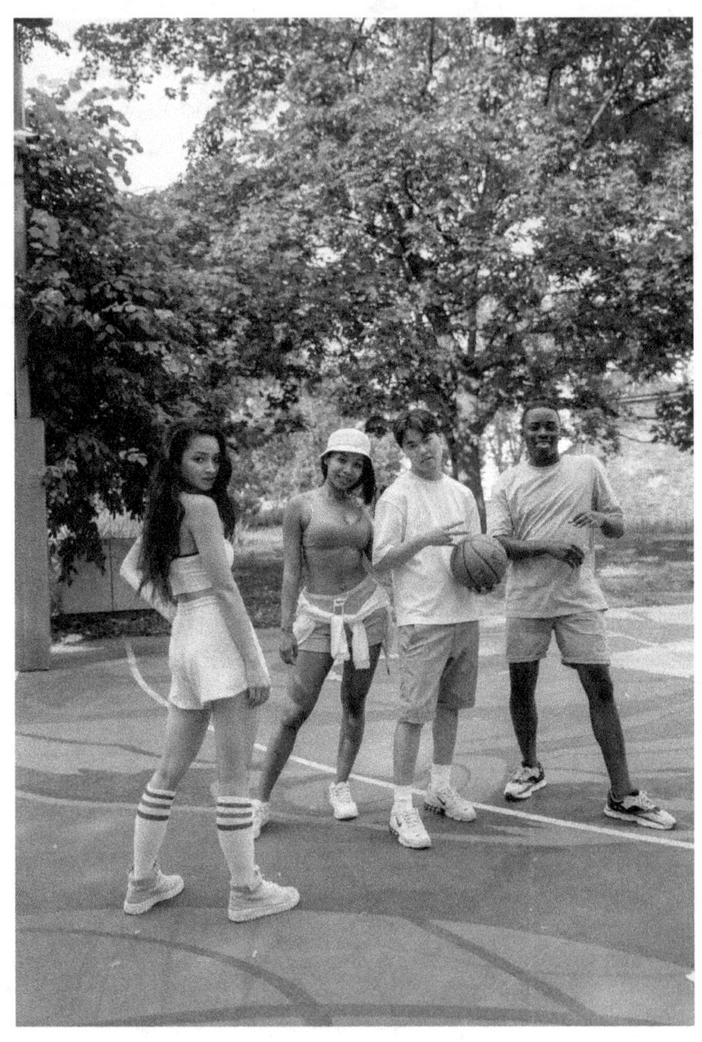

Chapter Six

VI. Putting It All Together: Creating Personalized Nutrition Plans

Creating a personalised nutrition plan involves integrating various elements tailored to an athlete's specific needs and goals:

1. Assess Individual Needs
Assessment: Understanding the athlete's sport, training regimen, goals, dietary preferences, and any specific health considerations.

Consultation:

Engaging with a qualified sports nutritionist or healthcare professional to assess nutritional requirements.

2. Establishing Baseline Nutrition
Baseline Diet: Designing a balanced diet rich in carbohydrates, proteins, healthy fats, vitamins, and minerals as the foundation.

Structuring meals and snacks around training schedules and competitions for optimal energy and recovery.

3. **Tailoring Nutritional Strategies Sport-Specific Needs:** Customising nutrition based on the demands of the athlete's specific sport or activity (e.g., endurance, strength, team sports).

Individual Factors:

Considering individual factors like age, gender, body composition, and any specific dietary intolerances or allergies.

4. **Incorporating Advanced Strategies Supplementation:** If deemed necessary, incorporate supplements cautiously under professional guidance to fill specific nutritional gaps.

Special Considerations:

Implementing advanced strategies for special populations (youth, older athletes) or focusing on mental performance when relevant.

5. Monitoring and Adjusting

Regular Evaluation: Periodically reassessing the plan's effectiveness, considering performance, recovery, and any changes in the athlete's goals or health status.

Adaptation:

Adjusting the nutrition plan as needed to optimise performance, recovery, and overall well-being.

By combining these elements and continuously adapting the plan based on individual responses and changing needs, a personalised nutrition plan can effectively support an athlete's performance goals while prioritising their health and long-term success.

A. Assessing Individual Needs

Assessing an athlete's individual needs involves a comprehensive evaluation to tailor a nutrition plan accordingly:

1. Sport-Specific Requirements

Understanding the Sport: Assessing the energy demands, duration, and intensity of the athlete's sport or activity.

Considering specific requirements based on the athlete's position or role in team sports or unique demands in individual sports.

2. Training and Competition Schedule

Training Load: Evaluating the frequency, duration, and intensity of training sessions to determine energy and nutrient needs.

Competition Timing:

Considering nutrition strategies specific to pre-, during, and post-competition periods for optimal performance.

3. Dietary Preferences and Restrictions

Preferences: Understanding the athlete's dietary preferences, including likes, dislikes, and cultural or ethical considerations.

Allergies or Intolerances:

Identifying any food allergies or intolerances to tailor the plan accordingly.

4. Body Composition and Goals

Body Composition: Assessing the athlete's body composition (muscle mass, body fat percentage) to determine nutritional requirements.

Performance Goals:

Understanding the athlete's goals, whether it's muscle gain, weight management, or specific performance improvements.

5. **Health and Medical History**
Medical Conditions: Considering any medical conditions or past injuries that might impact dietary choices or require specific nutritional modifications.

Medications:

Evaluating medications that may influence appetite, nutrient absorption, or have interactions with certain nutrients.

Gathering comprehensive information in these areas forms the foundation for creating a personalised nutrition plan that addresses the athlete's unique needs, supporting their performance goals while considering their overall health and well-being.

B. **Designing Customised Nutrition Plans for Performance Goals**

Designing customised nutrition plans for specific performance goals involves tailoring dietary strategies to meet the individual needs of the athlete. Here's a structured approach:

1. Define Performance Goals
Clarify Objectives: Clearly articulate the athlete's performance goals, whether it's strength gain, endurance improvement, weight management, or specific sport-related outcomes.

2. Energy Requirements
Calculate Energy Needs: Determine the athlete's daily caloric requirements based on factors such as basal metabolic rate, activity level, and specific training demands.

3. Macronutrient Distribution
Optimise Macronutrients: Adjust the distribution of carbohydrates, proteins, and fats based on the athlete's sport and performance goals. For example:
Endurance Sports: Prioritise carbohydrates for sustained energy.
Strength Training: Increase protein intake for muscle repair and growth.

4. Meal Timing Around Training Sessions
Pre-Exercise Nutrition: Tailor pre-exercise meals to provide adequate energy and support performance.

Intra-Exercise Nutrition: Consider strategies for fueling during prolonged activities if applicable.

Post-Exercise Nutrition:

Emphasise recovery with a combination of carbohydrates and proteins to replenish glycogen stores and aid muscle repair.

5. Hydration Strategies
Hydration Plan: Develop a personalised hydration strategy, considering factors like sweat rate, environmental conditions, and the duration of training or competition.

6. Micronutrient Considerations
Ensure Micronutrient Intake: Include a variety of fruits, vegetables, and whole grains to provide essential vitamins and minerals.

Supplementation if Necessary:

Consider supplementing specific nutrients if there are deficiencies or challenges in meeting requirements through food alone.

7. Monitoring and Adjusting
Regular Assessment: Periodically reassess the plan's effectiveness based on performance outcomes, energy levels, and overall well-being.

Adjustments: Make necessary adjustments to the nutrition plan as the athlete's goals, training regimen, or health status change.

By aligning nutrition strategies with specific performance objectives and continuously monitoring and adapting the plan, athletes can optimise their dietary approach to support their goals effectively. Working with a qualified sports nutritionist can provide valuable insights and guidance in this process.

C. **Tips for Sustainable and Consistent Nutrition Habits**

Absolutely, sustaining consistent nutrition habits is key for athletes to achieve long-term success. Here are some tips:

1. **Focus on Balanced and Varied Meals**

Diverse Diet: Emphasise a variety of nutrient-dense foods to ensure a wide spectrum of vitamins, minerals, and macronutrients.

Consistency: Strive for consistency in meal composition and timing to maintain energy levels throughout the day.

2. **Meal Preparation and Planning**

Meal Prepping: Plan and prepare meals ahead of time to ensure access to nutritious options during busy training or competition schedules.

Snack Choices: Have healthy snacks readily available to prevent impulse eating of less nutritious options.

3. Hydration as a Habit
Routine Hydration: Incorporate regular hydration habits into daily routines, aiming for consistent intake throughout the day.

Visual Cues: Use water bottles or hydration apps to track and ensure adequate daily fluid intake.

4. Gradual Changes and Flexibility
Gradual Adjustments: Implement changes in diet gradually rather than making drastic shifts, allowing for easier adaptation and sustainability.

Flexibility: Allow for occasional treats or deviations from the plan to maintain a healthy relationship with food and prevent feelings of restriction.

5. Education and Mindful Eating
Nutritional Knowledge: Continue learning about nutrition to make informed choices and better understand the impact of food choices on performance.

Mindful Eating: Practise mindful eating by focusing on hunger cues and savouring meals to enhance the eating experience and prevent overeating.

6. **Seek Professional Guidance and Support Consult Professionals:** Work with a registered dietitian or sports nutritionist to create a sustainable plan aligned with individual goals and needs.

Accountability and Support:

Joining a supportive community or having a training partner can aid in accountability and motivation for consistent nutrition habits.

Consistency in nutrition habits requires dedication, planning, and a balanced approach. By integrating these tips into their lifestyle, athletes can establish sustainable nutrition habits that support their long-term health and performance goals.

Chapter Seven

VII. Conclusion

In the world of sports and athletic performance, nutrition stands as a cornerstone for success. It's not just about fueling the body; it's a strategic approach to optimising performance, aiding recovery, and ensuring overall well-being.

Understanding the intricate connections between nutrition, energy, and athletic performance is pivotal. From the importance of macronutrients like carbohydrates, proteins, and fats to the role of micronutrients in enhancing performance, each element plays a vital part in an athlete's journey.

Tailoring nutrition plans to suit specific sports, activities, and individual needs allows athletes to unlock their full potential. Whether it's for endurance sports, strength and power training, or team sports, customised nutrition plans provide the necessary energy, nutrients, and hydration to excel.

Moreover, the broader considerations like mental performance, supplementation, and catering to special populations reflect the evolving landscape of sports nutrition. As research continues and knowledge expands, athletes can harness advanced strategies to fine-tune their nutrition plans, optimising both physical and mental aspects of their performance.

Ultimately, the key lies not just in devising a plan but in cultivating sustainable nutrition habits. Consistency, balance, and flexibility are the pillars that uphold these habits, ensuring they withstand the rigours of training, competition, and the demands of an athlete's life.

By embracing the principles of tailored nutrition, continual adaptation, and seeking professional guidance, athletes can pave their path toward sustained success, resilience, and peak performance, all supported by the power of optimal nutrition.

A. Recap: Key Takeaways for Optimising Performance Through Nutrition

Absolutely, here are the key takeaways to optimise performance through nutrition:

1. **Understanding Nutrient Needs Macronutrients:** Carbohydrates, proteins, and fats play essential roles in fueling workouts, aiding recovery, and supporting overall performance.

Micronutrients:

Vitamins and minerals are crucial for various bodily functions, including energy production and muscle function.

2. **Tailoring Nutrition to Sports and Activities**

Endurance Sports: Prioritise carbohydrates for sustained energy during long-duration activities like running or cycling.

Strength and Power Sports:

Increase protein intake to support muscle repair and growth after strength training.

Team Sports: Focus on fueling strategies for intermittent high-intensity activities and efficient recovery between games or matches.

3. **Optimal Timing and Hydration**

Pre-Exercise Fueling: Consume balanced meals or snacks pre-workout to ensure adequate energy levels.

Post-Exercise Nutrition:

Incorporate a blend of carbohydrates and proteins for glycogen replenishment and muscle recovery.

Hydration: Maintain consistent hydration habits, adjusting fluid intake based on activity levels and environmental conditions.

4. Supplementation and Individual Considerations

Supplements: Approach supplementation cautiously, seeking professional advice and considering individual needs and goals.

Special Populations:

Customise nutrition plans for youth and older athletes to support growth, development, and overall health.

5. Sustainable Nutrition Habits

Consistency: Aim for balanced and varied meals, consistent hydration, and gradual dietary adjustments for sustainability.

Planning and Preparation:

Plan meals ahead and have nutritious snacks readily available to maintain healthy eating habits.

6. Continuous Monitoring and Adaptation

Regular Evaluation: Periodically assess the nutrition plan's effectiveness based on performance outcomes and adjust as needed.

 Consult with registered dietitians or sports nutritionists for personalised advice and ongoing support.

By applying these key principles, athletes can create and maintain tailored nutrition plans that enhance their performance, aid recovery, and support overall health, ultimately contributing to their success in sports and athletic endeavours.

B. **The Future of Nutrition in Athletic Performance**

The future of nutrition in athletic performance is poised for exciting advancements and refinements. Here's what we might anticipate:

1. **Personalised Nutrition**
Genetic Insights: Leveraging genetic testing to tailor nutrition plans specific to an athlete's genetic makeup, optimising performance and health.

Precision Nutrition:

Using technology for precise tracking of individual responses to foods, enabling highly customised dietary recommendations.

2. Advanced Nutritional Strategies

Nutrigenomics: Exploring how specific nutrients interact with genes to impact athletic performance, recovery, and injury prevention.

Microbiome Research:

Understanding the role of gut health and its influence on nutrient absorption, immune function, and overall performance.

3. Technological Integration

Wearable Tech: Integrating data from wearable devices to personalise nutrition plans based on an athlete's real-time performance metrics.

Apps and Platforms:

Developing sophisticated apps or platforms for meal planning, tracking, and optimising nutrient intake tailored to athletes' needs.

4. Mind-Body Connection

Mental Performance Enhancement: Advancing the understanding of how nutrition impacts mental clarity, focus, and cognitive function for peak performance.

Holistic Approach:

Considering overall well-being, stress management, and sleep quality as integral parts of a comprehensive performance nutrition strategy.

5. **Sustainability and Ethical Considerations Environmental Impact:** Incorporating sustainable nutrition practices that reduce an athlete's ecological footprint without compromising performance.

Ethical Choices:

Addressing ethical considerations such as ethical sourcing of food and supplements aligned with an athlete's values and beliefs.

The future of sports nutrition holds promise in harnessing cutting-edge science, technology, and personalised approaches to optimise athletic performance while prioritising holistic health and sustainability. Integration of these advancements may revolutionise how athletes fuel their bodies, perform at their peak, and maintain long-term well-being.

VIII. Resources and References

Certainly! Here are some reputable resources and references for further exploration and reliable information on sports nutrition:

Websites and Organisations:
Academy of Nutrition and Dietetics (AND): Offers evidence-based resources and articles on sports nutrition.

Sports, Cardiovascular, and Wellness Nutrition (SCAN) Dietetic Practice Group: Provides specialised information and resources for sports nutrition professionals.

International Society of Sports Nutrition (ISSN):

Publishes scientific research, position stands, and guidelines on sports nutrition.

Books:
"Nancy Clark's Sports Nutrition Guidebook" by Nancy Clark: A comprehensive guide covering various aspects of sports nutrition.

"The Complete Guide to Sports Nutrition" by Anita Bean:

Explores nutrition for various sports, including meal plans and recipes.

Journals and Articles:

"Journal of the International Society of Sports Nutrition": Publishes peer-reviewed research articles on sports nutrition.

"Medicine & Science in Sports & Exercise" (MSSE):

Features studies and reviews on exercise physiology and nutrition.

Apps:
MyFitnessPal: Tracks nutrition, calories, and macros for meal planning and dietary analysis.

Cronometer: Helps track nutrient intake and provides detailed breakdowns of vitamins, minerals, and macros.

Registered Dietitians (RDs):

Consult with a certified sports dietitian or RD specialising in sports nutrition for personalised guidance.

Sports Nutritionists: Work with professionals specifically trained in sports nutrition for tailored advice and plans.

These resources offer credible information, research findings, and professional guidance to further explore and deepen understanding in the field of sports nutrition. Always prioritise reputable sources and consult with qualified professionals for personalised advice and recommendations.

Book Description

Fueling Peak Performance" is an authoritative and practical guide designed to empower athletes of all levels to optimise their nutrition for enhanced performance and overall well-being. Authored by a team of renowned sports nutritionists and registered dietitians, this comprehensive resource delves into the intricate relationship between nutrition and athletic excellence.

From understanding the fundamentals of macronutrients and micronutrients to tailoring nutrition plans for various sports and activities, this book offers a holistic approach. It explores the science behind energy metabolism, recovery strategies, and the impact of dietary choices on mental clarity and focus during training and competition.

Packed with evidence-based advice, meal plans, and recipes, "Fueling Peak Performance" provides actionable insights into:

Customising nutrition for specific sports, including endurance, strength, and team sports.
Precision meal planning around training sessions and competition timelines.
Advanced strategies like supplementation, micronutrient optimization, and genetic considerations for tailored nutrition plans.

Practical tips for sustainable eating habits, hydration strategies, and monitoring progress. Whether you're a beginner, elite athlete, or coach seeking to enhance performance through nutrition, this book serves as your definitive guide to unlock the potential of your body, fuel peak performance, and achieve your athletic goals.

This description highlights the comprehensive nature of the book, its focus on evidence-based advice, and its applicability for athletes across various levels and disciplines.

7 backend keyboards

1.Sports Nutrition Basics
2. Pre-Workout Nutrition
3. Post-Workout Recovery
4. Endurance Athlete Nutrition
5. Strength Training Nutrition
6. Hydration for Performance
7. Personalized Nutrition Plan

www.ingramcontent.com/pod-product-compliance
Lightning Source LLC
Chambersburg PA
CBHW070800250726
48662CB00004B/1904